3
Cholesterol Cure

LIVE LONGER AND HEALTHIER BY LOWERING YOUR CHOLESTEROL NATURALLY

Brought To You By:

C.J. Walker

INTRODUCTION

I want to thank you and congratulate you for downloading, *"30 Day Cholesterol Cure"*.
This book contains proven steps and strategies on how to fight cholesterol using natural dietary methods without any dangerous statin drugs.

This guide will help you understand what cholesterol is, why it elevates, and how to lower cholesterol naturally and safely.

If you're reading this book, probably you or someone you care about has been diagnosed with "high cholesterol" from a medical professional. But having a diagnosis of "high cholesterol" and knowing what it is or how it got there can be two different things.

It's also important to know that you can treat high cholesterol naturally!

In today's world pharmaceutical drugs are prescribed far too readily. While prescription drugs may treat the symptoms very quickly, they don't address the underlying issues on what caused the problem in the first place. So even though your symptoms may be under control you still have a problem!

In addition, pharmaceutical drugs often have side effects that can compromise other aspects of your health and eventually leave you worse off than when you started.

On the other hand, the strategies you will learn about in this book are all-natural and proven to work! Imagine not having to take cholesterol meds ever again...or ever having to start in the first place! That's exciting isn't it? I'm excited for you because the information contained in this book can literally change your health forever!

Enjoy the book,
C.J. Walker

P.S. If you do enjoy the book please leave a review on Amazon!

DISCLAIMER:

These exercise and nutrition ideas are for information purposes only. The information presented is in no way intended as medical advice or to serve as a substitute for medical counseling. The information should be used in conjunction with the guidance and care of your physician.

By utilizing the exercise and/or nutrition strategies contained herein, you recognize that despite all precautions on the part of the author there are risks of injury or illness that can occur as with any nutrition/exercise program.

You assume all risks and waive, relinquish, and release any claim to which you may have against the author or any other related parties in the event of any physical injury or illness incurred in connection with, or as a result of, the use or misuse of the information contained on these pages.

What the heck is cholesterol anyway?

Cholesterol is a fatty and wax-like substance that belongs to the steroids class of lipids. It is present in all the body cells and is synthesized mainly in the liver. It can also be taken from the food; in fact most of the excess fats are the result of some diets. I call it a double-edge sword since it is both-our friend and enemy. It is essentially required for some of the crucial body functions and at the same time, it can evoke a heart attack when present in abnormally increased quantities. It is an important factor in estimating the risk of stroke or heart attack in an individual.

Types of cholesterol:

Since cholesterol is a subclass of lipids it does not dissolve in the blood, which is mainly water. This oil-based substance attaches to certain proteins and then this compound gets circulated in the blood. This cholesterol and protein combination is termed as lipoprotein. The types of lipoproteins are based on the percentage of proteins and fat in the combination. The cholesterol carrying proteins are:

Low density lipoproteins (LDLs): Low density lipoproteins are known as 'bad cholesterol' owing to their tendency of causing plaque on the arteries, thereby increasing the risk of stroke and heart attack.

High density lipoproteins (HDLs): The cholesterol attached to these proteins is not harmful for the body so this form of cholesterol is considered 'good cholesterol'. It helps to reduce the LDLs; hence it's good for you to have a higher level of HDL.

Very low density lipoproteins (VLDLs): This kind is very similar to low density lipoproteins and is high in lipid content.

Triglycerides: This is the storage form of cholesterol. Alcohol, sugar and an excess of calories are converted into triglycerides and are stored in cells.

THE GOOD ASPECTS OF CHOLESTEROL:

As I said earlier, cholesterol is essential to live. It is the modulator of many important metabolic reactions. Cholesterol is so important that we cannot survive without its normal amounts. The major functions of cholesterol in our body are:

1. Cell membrane integrity:

Cholesterol produces and maintains the cell membrane, which is crucial for sustaining life. Any kind of damage to cell membrane integrity leads to serious consequences, and cholesterol provides a stable structure to the cell membrane. This is the most important function that allows the cell substances to remain in their limited locations.

2. Vitamin D production:

Cholesterol acts as parent substances and helps the body produce vitamin D with the exposure to sunlight or ultraviolet rays.

3. Bile production:

Cholesterol makes the bile salts that help in digestion and absorption.

4. Hormones production:

Cholesterol acts as a source compound, enabling the body to reduce certain steroidal hormones such as estrogen, testosterone, cortisol, progesterone and aldosterone.

WHAT ARE THE NORMAL BODY CHOLESTEROL LEVELS?

It is recommended that everyone gets their cholesterol checked every fifth year after the age of 20 years old. Since high cholesterol does not produce any symptoms, it is considered a "silent killer". The only way to determine the cholesterol level is by getting it analyzed.

There are fasting and non-fasting tests to determine the levels of different types of cholesterol. A non-fasting test measures the total cholesterol and HDL, while a fasting test will measure the LDL, HDL, triglycerides and total cholesterol. Below are the quantities that are used to determine the normality of cholesterol and the risk of heart attack.

HDL amounts:
- High: 60 mg/dL or above.
- Low: below 40 mg/dL

LDL amounts:
- Very high: 190 mg/dL and above.
- High: 160 to 189 mg/dL
- Near-optimal: 100 to 129 mg/dL
- Optimal: less than 100 mg/dL

Total cholesterol values:
- High: 240 mg/dL or above.
- Desirable: less than 200 mg/dL

FACTORS AFFECTING CHOLESTEROL LEVEL:

There are a number of factors that can alter the amount cholesterol in the body. Some of the factors affect the synthesis of cholesterol, while others take part in the process of its utilization. Below is a list of main factors that are important in determining cholesterol levels in a person.

1. Genetics: Hereditary factors are important as a person may have inherited the high cholesterol genes from his/her parents. Hence, the problem of high cholesterol can run in families.

2. Age: Cholesterol increases as we get older.

3. Gender: Gender is not an extremely important determining factor; however, it is seen that women can have increased levels of LDL after menopause as compared to men of same age.

4. Diet: Taking in high amounts of saturated fats and high cholesterol foods regularly can increase cholesterol. We will be describing the details on cholesterol and your diet in the subsequent chapters.

5. Exercise: Active people have decreased chances of having abnormal cholesterol levels as their bodies utilize it better. Regular exercise can decrease the HDL and LDL too.

6. Medical conditions: There are certain medical conditions that can cause high cholesterol in body. Diabetes is one of the most common conditions that can contribute to higher cholesterol. Poorly controlled diabetes disturbs the metabolism and you may get an elevated cholesterol level.

FORGET ABOUT DANGEROUS STATIN DRUGS

Tens of millions of Americans are taking some sort of drug to help control high cholesterol. Most of these drugs being what are called "statins".

What are statin drugs?

Statins are a group of drugs that act on the liver cell receptors and block the formation of cholesterol. These inhibit the precursor fat molecules that are necessary for making cholesterol. Statins were designed to treat the fatal diseases like angina, atherosclerosis and heart attacks. These are also prescribed for morbid obesity. Some of the available statin drugs are Advicor, Altoprev, Caduet, Crestor, Lescol, Lipitor, Mevacor, Pravachol, Simcor and Zocor. Yes, statin drugs may be useful in some very lethal situations in the short term, but that's not how these drugs are generally prescribed.

How statin drugs work:

HMG_CoA Reductase enzyme is required for the production of cholesterol in the liver. The statins mimic the HMG_CoA reductase and binds to its receptors thereby replacing this enzyme. This blocks the production of cholesterol.

Why should you avoid statin drugs?

As the chapter name says, we recommend you not to consider statin drugs as they can wreak havoc on your body. The ability to tolerate statins varies from person to person, but the side effects are so numerous that everyone is affected in the end. Some of the common side effects are:

- Dizziness
- Drowsiness
- Headache
- Insomnia *(inability to sleep)*
- Flushing of skin
- Muscle pain
- Tenderness and generalized weakness
- Nausea and vomiting
- Bloating
- Diarrhea
- Abdominal cramps
- Constipation

Above are some common side effects that appear with the usage of statin drugs. These effects are not fatal and can be tolerated. However, statins do exert some life threatening effects that can culminate in a medical emergency. Some of the potentially lethal effects of statins are:

a. Liver damage:

Statins interact with other chemicals in the liver and can increase the liver enzymes. This increase may be mild or severe. It is recommended to check the level of liver enzymes while taking the statin drugs.

b. Muscle problems like myositis:

Myositis is inflammation or swelling of the muscles. There's a direct correlation between the statin drugs and the level of pain you'll feel from the inflammation of your muscle tissue. The higher the dosage, the more intense the muscle pain.

c. Type-2 diabetes:

The increased blood sugar levels due to use of statins may give rise to type-2 diabetes mellitus.

d. Neurological problems:

Although there is little evidence of major neurological problems, there are still chances of neurological damage due to statin drugs. According to the FDA, statins are linked with memory loss and states of confusion.

e. Elevated levels of CK (creatine kinase):

Creatine kinase is a muscle enzyme that should be present in a limited amount. Statins can increase its level, and it will ultimately cause pain and inflammation.

f. Rhabdomyolysis:

This is the condition of extreme muscular damage caused by statins where muscles become tender, weak and painful all over the body. Rhabdomyolysis is the breakdown of muscle fibers that leads to the release of the muscle fiber contents (myoglobin) into the bloodstream. Myoglobin is harmful to the kidneys and often causes kidney damage. There is a risk of renal failure and death when there is severe rhabdomyolysis.

Since these are very serious effects and may even cause the death of the patient, we definitely recommend that you don't consider these drugs as your first option to cure your cholesterol problems. We highly suggest using the strategies you are about to learn to get your cholesterol under control, naturally, first before getting started with any of these dangerous medications. In severe circumstances your doctor may require you to start a medication but your goal should be to follow the steps outlined in this book and work with your doctor to wean yourself off of the statin drug(s) as soon as possible!

IS CHOLESTEROL REALLY THAT BAD? BREAKING THE BAD CHOLESTEROL MYTH...

Before proceeding to the foods and other measures of reducing cholesterol, it is necessary to clear up some confusion about cholesterol. Whenever I look at the news, print, or social media, all I see is the negative side of the media portraying cholesterol as all bad. From health and wellness personalities to the pharmaceutical industry, it is a common trend to label the cholesterol as something completely negative. However, we must not forget the vital role of cholesterol in maintaining our body and sustaining life.

Cholesterol is vital and is a 'good thing' in our bodies. As we previously mentioned, cholesterol is necessary for many functions in the body, such as the digestion of our food all the way to our neurological functions.

Inflammation is the main culprit in many instances that not only tends to deposit the cholesterol on arteries but also breaks the continuity of vessel walls. In response to inflammatory process, cholesterol plays a protective role in most of these instances. However, when damage is extensive and cholesterol deposits are high, then it leads to the narrowing of the arteries and increases the risk of stroke and heart attack.

Moderate increases in cholesterol are not life-threatening; however, if cholesterol levels exceed a certain level, then you most definitely have a serious health situation. All the possible measures should be taken to keep it within normal amounts. This reiterates the importance of getting your cholesterol checked periodically to ensure that your diet and lifestyle are helping you maintain healthy levels, as there are no outward signs of high cholesterol.

9 Foods to Never Eat If you Have High Cholesterol

Diet is the main source of accumulated cholesterol in the body. Diet can either cure or further aggravate the cholesterol problem. In this section, we will describe both the bad (increasing cholesterol) and good (reducing cholesterol) foods to give you an idea about what to take and what to avoid.

FOODS THAT ARE HIGH IN CHOLESTEROL:

The foods containing saturated fats are the main dietary cause of elevated cholesterol levels. Most of these high fat foods are obtained from animal sources. People who consume animal products in abundance without the proper balance of nutrients in their diet (i.e. fresh fruits, vegetables etc...) have been seen to have increased risk of higher cholesterol. It is observed that people who consume a primarily plant-based diet are less likely to get high cholesterol as their dietary intake of cholesterol is minimum. Below are a few examples of foods that contain dangerous levels of saturated fat:

- Ghee
- Butter
- Lard
- Hard margarines
- Dairy fats

The above mentioned products are saturated fats or 'unhealthy' fats so these must be consumed in moderation, or even limited quantities. Saturated fats tend to accumulate more than the unsaturated ones.

Below are 9 of the highest cholesterol containing foods:

1. Egg yolk

A single egg yolk provides 210mg of cholesterol that is highest among the other foods. People who already have an increased fatty level should avoid yolks. The egg white is rich in protein and is great for your diet.

2. Fish roe:

It is commonly used with bread in European countries and is very rich in cholesterol. 100 grams of fish roe contains 588mg of cholesterol, making it about 100mg per tablespoon.

3. Liver:

The liver is the factory of cholesterol synthesis so it makes sense that liver cells are filled with cholesterol. 100 grams of liver contains about 565mg of cholesterol.

4. Butter:

Butter is a saturated fat that is used in almost every place in the world. It's flavor is undeniably rich and delicious on bread, cakes, vegetables etc...But it should definitely be consumed in moderation. 100

grams of butter contains about 215 mg of cholesterol.

5. Fast foods:

We all know that fast food is not healthy food. It is some of the most processed, fatty, fried, and junk-filled "food" you can eat. To have a healthy body we must abstain from these killer foods.

6. Shrimp:

A large shrimp contains about 50 mg of cholesterol, placing it among high cholesterol foods.

7. Cheese:

Another commonly used high cholesterol food that contains 25mg per one inch cube.

8. Shellfish:

Shellfish are eaten in a variety of forms: powdered, raw, fried or steamed. 100 grams of shellfish contains about 110 mg of cholesterol.

9. Processed meats:

These foods are highly rich in cholesterol and because they are processed (not naturally occurring) they can lead to other health issues, beside increased cholesterol.

However, there are some other food choices that may not be very rich in cholesterol but their continuous consumption can have a notable impact on your cholesterol levels. You may also be surprised by looking at this list as these are not generally associated with an increased affect on cholesterol levels.

Moderate your intake of the following "moderate" cholesterol foods:

- Snack crackers, muffins
- Added sugars
- Turkey
- Pizza
- Mashed potatoes
- Coconut oil
- Whole fats dairy products
- Pastries and pie
- Butter-drenched or sugar-coated popcorn, candies, etc...

A healthy person whose cholesterol is "healthy" or within range can consume many of the above mentioned foods in moderation. However, a person with elevated cholesterol should definitely make his/her best efforts to avoid these foods and focus on their nutrition.

TOP 7 CHOLESTEROL LOWERING FOODS

After having the discussion about cholesterol rich foods, we'll now touch on the foods that are, not only low in cholesterol, but also have the ability to decrease the cholesterol in the body by decreasing its absorption and increasing its excretion. We suggest whole, unprocessed foods in your diet so that you can reap the benefits of lowering your cholesterol naturally. Here are the top 7 cholesterol lowering foods:

1. Oats:

Oats are one of the best foods to help lower your cholesterol naturally. Oats contain beta glucan, which is a type of soluble fiber. It binds to the walls of digestive tract and form a layer that prevents the absorption of cholesterol and it is excreted from body. 3 grams of beta glucan per day are sufficient to produce this cholesterol excretion effect. Oats are an important source of daily fiber (most adults should aim for 25-35 grams of fiber per day). So start making healthy, delicious oats a part of your regular routine!

2. Olive oil:

Olive oil is a healthy oil as it contains unsaturated fats which help to control cholesterol. It strengthens the arteries and provides the body enough time to get rid of extra fats. Try to use at least two tablespoons of olive oil into your daily routine. Try drizzling a tablespoon of oil over your veggies for a rich yummy flavor, and great dose of healthy fats!

3. Beans:

"Beans, Beans, the magical fruit..." – We've all heard the tune right!? It turns out that beans really are magical when it comes to reducing LDL cholesterol. Beans are full of fiber which helps reduce the LDL cholesterol from you blood. So try and add at least 1 serving of beans to your diet regimen daily.

4. Nuts:

Nuts are rich in many valuable nutrients such as plant sterols, fiber, mono-unsaturated fats and vitamin E. Even eating as few as 10 nuts in a day are sufficient to produce healthy effects in your body. Our recommended dose for nuts is 50g per day.

5. Fiber:

Fiber is found in many foods (vegetables, beans, whole grains etc...) It binds to cholesterol in your gut and is excreted in waste. As we mentioned earlier, 25-35 grams of fiber is recommended for your daily intake to keep your body running efficiently.

6. Fish:

Fish contains a high level of omega-3 fatty acids. Omega 3's are essential for a healthy heart and blood vessels. It has the additional benefit of reducing blood pressure and preventing the clot formation within the vessels. Our recommended dose is at least 2 servings of fish in a week.

7. Avocados:

Avocados are another great source of health fats! Avocados are high in oleic acid which not only lowers the bad cholesterol (LDL) but it also raises the good cholesterol. A great way to incorporate avocados into your diet is to make up some fresh guacamole dip to keep in the refrigerator and add 1-2 tablespoons to one of your meals each day.

TOP 3 SUPPLEMENTS FOR MANAGING CHOLESTEROL NATURALLY

1. Fish Oil

Fish oil contains an abundance of omega 3 fatty acids (healthy fat) which have been proven to lower triglycerides, reduce inflammation and protect against a variety of conditions like heart attack and stroke. If you can't get enough healthy fats through your diet then supplementing with fish oil is good idea. A good dose to start with is 2-4 grams per day. If you have a problem with "fishy burps" try getting capsules that are "enteric coated" or have lemon oil added to them. *If you taking a blood thinner make sure to let your doctor know you're starting a fish oil supplement.

2. Multi-vitamin

I shouldn't have to tell you to take a multi-vitamin but I'm going to anyway because so many people don't. The fact is that if you're having high cholesterol issues they most likely stem from not eating the right foods. If you're not eating the right foods I can all but guarantee you're not getting the vitamins and minerals your body needs to function at an optimal level. Research also shows us that even if you are eating a "healthy diet" that we often don't get the vitamins and minerals we need due to several factors including: nutrient depletion from the soil and/or lack of variety in our diets.

3. Vitamin D3

Vitamin D3 is actually more like a hormone in terms of how it acts in the body. It is vitally important to help maintain a healthy immune system, strong bones and a positive mental outlook. Studies also show us that vitamin D3 reduces heart disease, osteoporosis, depression, cancer, helps with weight loss issues and more! It's safe to say that most people should supplement with an additional 1-2,000 iu of vitamin D3 daily, but people that are taking statin drugs or have taken statin drugs may want to consider higher doses. Statins can actually decrease the amount of D3 your body's able to manufacture naturally which can leave you open to all sorts of health issues long term. You can have your vitamin D3 levels checked at your doctor very inexpensively and adjust your dosages accordingly.

TOP 10 HERBS TO MANAGE CHOLESTEROL NATURALLY

In addition to all the foods we talked about to help control and lower cholesterol, we also want to talk about the ten amazing herbs that specifically help lower cholesterol naturally. These herbs are not only beneficial in helping lower cholesterol, but they add variety to your food & taste great!

1. Psyllium:

Regarding cholesterol, it has been established that ingesting about 5 grams of psyllium, twice a day, causes a notable reduction in both the low density lipoproteins and total serum cholesterol.

2. Capsicum:

This spicy herb is commonly used in chilies and salsas. The ingredients of this herb improve the blood flow and reduce the possibility of blood clotting. A connection between capsicum and lowered cholesterol levels has been established by many research studies.

3. Butcher's Broom:

Butcher's Broom increases the blood circulation to extremities, strengthens the arteries, relaxes the vessels and prevents degeneration of arterial tissue.

4. Guggul:

Guggul also reduces the triglycerides in addition to LDL. It contains many useful ingredients such as resin, gum and volatile oils that perform cleansing functions.

5. Hawthorn Berry:

Like capsicum, this herb also exerts many beneficial effects on heart health. It relaxes and smoothes the blood vessels, decreases the chances of vessels' degeneration, and increases the blood flow to extremity tissues.

6. Red yeast rice:

Red yeast rice has been shown to be helpful in achieving the goal of cholesterol loss. It is also a part of many over the counter cholesterol decreasing supplements.

7. Fenugreek seeds:

This herb contains alkaloids and lysine; both have the qualities of decreasing LDLs without any side effects.

8. Licorice root:

Licorice root has a protective effect on blood vessels and stabilizes the heart rhythm.

9. Policosanol:

Policicosanol is extracted from sugar cane and has been known to reduce cholesterol. However, it hasn't been exactly determined how policosanol works in the body to reduce cholesterol.

10. Garlic:

Garlic has been used since for many centuries in cultures all across the globe. In addition to adding wonderful flavor to foods, it has a number of health benefits. It has been shown to decrease the serum cholesterol. It also strengthens the vessels and decreases the blood clotting. Work in 2-3 cloves of fresh garlic daily for optimal health and cholesterol reduction.

CAN GREEN TEA FIX YOUR CHOLESTEROL?

Green tea has become a celebrity of sorts in the health world due to its extensive literature and publicity in health magazines, the news, & social media. Does it deserve it? My answer is yes. Green tea has been a part of traditional medicine for centuries. Unlike many other alternative drugs, green tea has complied with scientific studies and is also endorsed by doctors. It has a variety of health benefits that go beyond helping reduce cholesterol, but that's where our focus will be today: on reducing cholesterol.

According to the American Journal of Clinical Nutrition (2011), it was proved by scientific analysis that people who consumed more green tea had lower levels of LDL or 'bad' cholesterol. It was seen that levels of HDL or 'good' cholesterol were not affected by it. Since green tea is rich in many polyphenolic components, the exact component responsible for cholesterol decrease has not yet been pinpointed.

How is green tea different from other tea products? The biggest difference is less processing. Green tea undergoes much less processing and refinement as compared to other teas and tea products. Because of this lack of processing, the antioxidants of green tea are preserved and its benefits are much more potent. Catechins are the most important among the antioxidants in green tea. Let's talk about how green tea helps to reduce cholesterol.

HOW DOES IT WORK?

According to many research studies, it is found that green tea components inhibit the enzymes that are needed for cholesterol synthesis. There are 6 different catechins in green tea. ECG and EGCG are the two most potent ones and provide the healing properties of green tea.

There are also some additional effects that make it a potent fat shredder. It helps to suppress appetite, burns fat and accelerates the metabolic rate.

HOW MUCH TEA IS NEEDED DAILY?

You'll probably hear nutritionists giving several different opinions on the quantity of green tea you should drink every day. However, **most experts advise 4 cups per day to reap all of the health benefits, including lowering your cholesterol.** Don't drink too much tea close to bedtime as it can affect your sleep because of its naturally occurring caffeine content. It's also important to note that you get your green tea from a reputable source. The most ideal is to go organic with your green tea.

How to Make Iced Green Tea

Does drinking 4 cups of green tea daily sound overwhelming? Drinking iced green tea is an easy way to get in your 4 cups daily since you can drink it cold and get more tea in at once. It's also very easy to make!

Step 1: Boil 6-7 cups of hot water
Step 2: Place 3-4 bags of green tea into a BPA free plastic container or glass container
Step 3: Pour hot water into your container
Step 4: Add 1-2 cups of ice
Step 5: Place container in refrigerator until cold

Want more flavor in your green tea? Here are a few ways to sweeten up your tea and add more flavor:

- If you like your green tea a little bit sweeter you can add "stevia" & sweeten to your

liking. *(Stevia is an all natural, plant-derived, 0 calorie sweetener)*
- Try adding fresh mint leaves
- Add lemon or lime wedges

DIET FOR HIGH CHOLESTEROL

Now that you have a good idea of which foods to eat and which foods to stay away from I want to give you an outline of what a sample day might look like. This is designed to be an outline rather than giving specific recipes as you will probably want some variety in your life, right? Plus there are plenty of great recipes online that you can use that fit within these guidelines!

BREAKFAST IDEAS

Vitamins/Supplements
Green tea or large glass of lemon water
+
Egg white omelet with 1-2 cups chopped veggies and salsa
or
Oatmeal with fresh berries + Scrambled egg whites

LUNCH IDEAS

Vitamins/Supplements
Green tea or large glass of lemon water

+
Ezekiel tortilla wrap with 4-6oz chicken, black beans and guacamole
or
Salad with 4-6oz chicken, chopped veggies, oil and vinegar

Dinner Ideas

Vitamins/Supplements
Green tea or large glass of lemon water
+
4-6 oz salmon with 2-3 cups of steamed veggies
Or
Halibut with asparagus

Walking to reduce cholesterol

Walking and increasing your daily "step" count is crucial for your general health and helping to maintain a healthy weight. It prevents and cures many disorders and is the most healthy activity that keeps us active and disease free. It affects our body from head to toe in a positive way. The extra activity level you receive from walking is also effective in lowering the cholesterol levels.

Walking is an aerobic exercise and decreases the cholesterol by burning fat and reducing stress. According to a U.S. cholesterol program, walking on a regular basis is one of the most powerful ways to help rid your body of "bad" cholesterol.

We have two walking plans based on your age. **If you are 30-50 years of age, we recommend that you walk about 2 miles three times a week, and try to increase that number until it becomes 2 miles daily. For people who are 50 years of age or older, we recommend that you walk one mile four times per week, and then gradually increase your walking to 2 miles four times per week.**

Walking Tips:

- Try to have a partner or some company as you take your walk. It will keep you motivated and you won't get bored or tired of walking. Instead walking can become a fun, healthy daily ritual.
- Put down your car keys and try to walk instead of drive whenever possible. If your office or college is near, walk there! Walk whenever possible, even if it's just walking across the street to the market or meeting up with a friend. Pretty soon it will be no big deal to get in that daily two mile walk!
- Watch your posture as you walk. Improper posture can cause damage to your body. So stand up tall, shoulders back, and enjoy that walk!
- Don't overdo it. Start with a small distance and increase it slowly. Stop when you are tired or if you become overheated.
- Don't be afraid to take a small break here and there to catch your breath. Plus, make sure to hydrate with water before and after your walk. If you want to carry a water

bottle you can definitely take it with you on your walk to refresh yourself.
- Is it sub-arctic weather outside? Or is over 100 degree outside? No problem. You can always invest in a treadmill, or for a cheaper option you walk around your home. It may seem silly, but it is walking just the same whether it is inside or outside. Many people also enjoy going to the local shopping mall during inclement weather to get in their daily walk!
- Put on some tunes. Listening to music does so many great things for your health & mind. So put on your headphones and get walking!

CONCLUSION:

Thank you for choosing this book to help you learn how to lower your cholesterol naturally. I really hope that you have found value within these pages. We've covered both the science behind fixing your cholesterol and the practical strategies you can use to start lowering your cholesterol right away.

To your health,

C.J. Walker

P.S. If you have found value in this book please leave me a great review on Amazon! I want to reach as many people as possible with the message of health and wellness!